10
LITTLE RULES
OF HANK

One family's journey
through a rare disease

by Wendy Price

ISBN-13: 978-0-9974799-2-8

For more information visit www.10littlerules.com

dedication

To Jamey, my husband and best friend;
you are the sole reason for my sanity. Thank you.

To Hank and Dave, my two very favorite little guys.
Everyday is a good day with you two in it.

And to all kids who have been diagnosed
with a rare disease, and their families.

We are all one family – stay strong.
We've got this.

table of contents

foreword   11

introduction   13

rule #1 - wake up   15

rule #2 - lose the guilt   23

rule #3 - don't panic; get a plan   31

rule #4 - don't become a prisoner   41

rule #5 - forward your thoughts   49

rule #6 - redefine normal   57

rule #7 - seek out others   65

rule #8 - embrace the humor   75

rule #9 - make it better   83

rule #10 - every day, give thanks   93

rule #11 - carry on...   101

Table of Contents

foreword

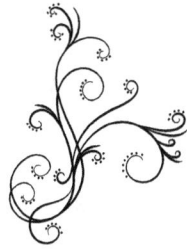

Wendy Price is one of those rare women you meet in the world who always takes things to the next level. She has a massive heart and an astonishingly low tolerance for BS. To the people in her life, this makes her a superhero, loving with everything she's got, and taking no prisoners when it comes to protecting her own.

Wendy left a career she loved to work from home and care for her young sons when her youngest, Hank, was diagnosed with a medical condition that makes life … a bit interesting … for the whole family. We welcome Wendy to the 10 Little Rules family, and are thrilled that she's chosen to share her family's story with our community. We wish her and her beautiful, amazing family every good thing as they journey forward together.

10 Little Rules is a community of people, books, advice, support and love, created to help us all find that little something that will make our lives flow a bit better. Wendy, Hank and her entire family belong here, and I am honored to introduce them to you.

Carol Pearson
Founder, 10 Little Rules
www.10littlerules.com

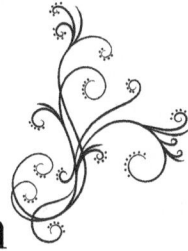

introduction

There is no way for me to give you any tips or rules for getting through a rare diagnosis without sharing our family's story of Hank.

My youngest child became known as "The Puker" at his day care. He wasn't sick, but after nearly every meal he'd throw up. No temperature, no cries of pain beforehand, no discernible rhyme or rhythm.

The puking got so bad the caretakers in his room began to bring in a change of clothing. There was no warning, and no way to predict when it would happen.

We took Hank to the pediatrician; we were told it was a stomach virus. Two weeks later, it was acid reflux. The search for answers continued.

Our pediatrician was amazing with medical puzzles. He asked us about the actual vomit itself, as well as, was is projectile? Did it happen immediately after eating? Was his head spinning around and was split pea soup showering all over those who were near? Ok, he didn't ask that last one, but there were days when my husband and I could answer that with a resounding "YES!"

He dropped a comment that made us think we might be dealing with something called "EoE." We didn't have a clue what "EoE" meant but this was the day we started on our journey of discovery. Discovery of what it was, what causes it, what it means for Hank, and how on earth to manage it. This, it turned out, is about as easy as asking a toddler to clean up after himself; living with trial and error, with the guidance and support of our pediatrician, became our new normal.

Regardless of what rare illness your family is dealing with, many of the steps along the journey are the same. Your emotions and frustrations are the same. Whether it's EoE like my son, or another disease, we are the same.

We are all scared, we are all tired and heartbroken and, as such, we are going through this together. I hope that sharing our story and the rules we use to move forward will help you move forward as well.

Wendy

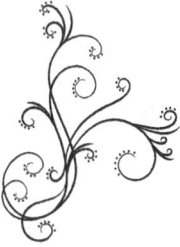

RULE #1
wake up

With two kids in daycare and working 40-plus hours a week, my husband and I were going crazy. We didn't know what was causing our youngest to vomit after each meal. We didn't understand why his cradle cap didn't go away, no matter what we tried, or why Hank's full body rashes seemed to be getting worse. We just didn't understand.

We didn't have time for the seemingly nonstop doctor's appointments, or the patience for being told that it was just a virus and eczema and we needed to give him Tylenol and slather him down with lotion.

We were at our wits' end. We could no longer take the family out for a sit-down dinner, the Tylenol wasn't working and the lotion seemed to sting, even though we were using baby lotions for sensitive skin. Something more was going on here.

We WOKE UP. We knew his symptoms were not coming from a virus. We started keeping lists of what he ate and calendars of when he vomited. We monitored his rashes and experimented with new homemade lotions; we gave him oatmeal baths from organic steel oats that I ground myself at home (which, for the record, ended in a full body rash). Most importantly, we requested an allergy test from his pediatrician. We didn't know if he had allergies; between my husband and I, we only have a few. We live in Michigan, so we also have

15

RULE #1
Wake Up

trouble with pollen, like nearly everyone else here in the Mitten State. We simply had no idea what was going on and decided this was a logical step. The findings were a blow to our family.

When the nurse called to go over the results, I was just leaving the office to pick up my boys from daycare. She told me to turn around because I was going to need to sit down and write it all down.

Hank was allergic to wheat, egg whites, barley, sesame, tree and peanuts, dairy and oranges, and we needed to pick up an EpiPen right away from the pharmacy. We were also given a warning: There may be more foods that he is allergic to and blood testing wasn't conclusive. How scary is that, to have a list of items read out to you and be told there are likely more?!?

After another pediatrician appointment we found ourselves with a possible diagnosis (that mysterious EoE was mentioned again), and a referral to a pediatric gastrointestinal specialist as well as an allergist.

After an endoscopy, it was confirmed. My beautiful two-year-old baby, Hank, had a rare autoimmune disease: Eosinophilic Esophagitis, or EoE for short.

In simple terms, Hank's body is allergic to food and his environment; his reactions included the vomiting, hives (the ones around his mouth were the start of an anaphylactic reaction), and itching. Reactions could be as severe as food impaction or worse.

Waking up, while terrifying, had an unexpected and amazing benefit. Oddly, it brought a measure of relief. Suddenly, I started feeling as though we could handle whatever came our way, now that we knew what we were dealing with. We knew we had to start thinking outside of our comfort zone, but we also knew we'd somehow be able to do that. Together, we knew we'd be able to move forward.

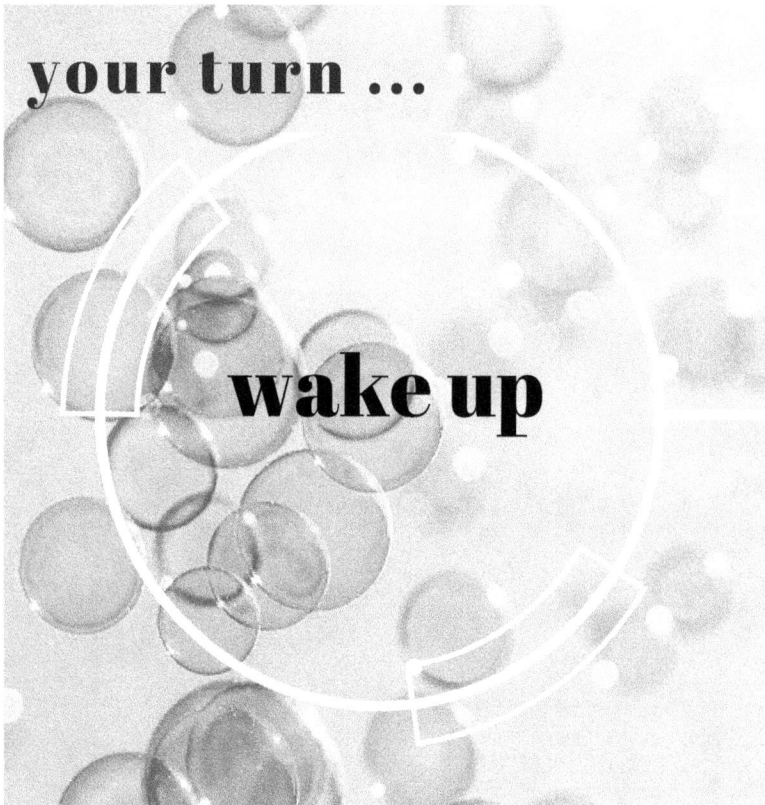

your turn ...

wake up

Take some time and honestly evaluate your new situation. Start organizing your thoughts on the next few pages. Write down what is happening and what your instinct tells you to do to move forward. Do you need another doctor's opinion? Do you need to speak to a hospital support specialist? Do you need a better understanding of new medications? Write it all down here; your thoughts don't need to be in order, they just need to be written down. Trust your gut.

1

wake up

date _____

date _____

wake up

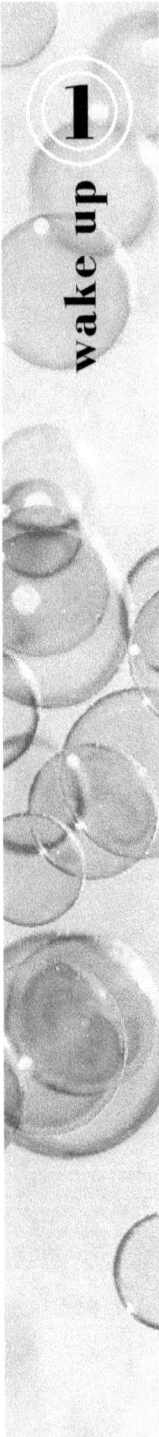

1

wake up

date _____

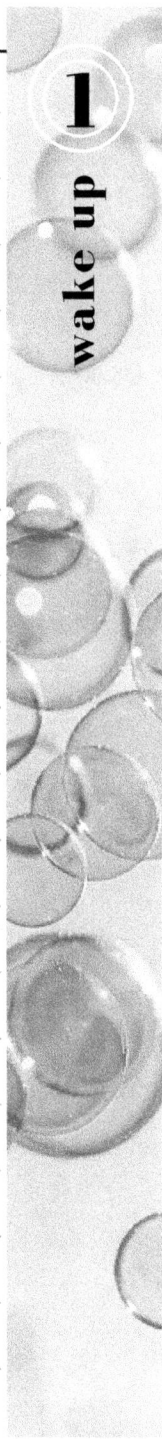

date _____

wake up

1

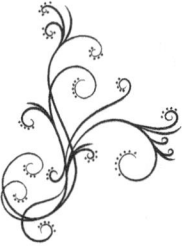

RULE #2
lose the guilt

After his EoE diagnosis, one of the hardest parts of moving forward was coming to terms with how Hank came to have this condition; I felt guilty that maybe I had passed this genetic condition to my baby. Since the diagnosis, it's come to light that some of the issues that I have had with food and the environment points to me having EoE as well.

Hank's allergist did tell us that I passed this down genetically. Was it my fault? Was I a horrible person for doing this to my child?

No.

I have two children; Dave was and remains a healthy child with an appetite to rival any large carnivore. He doesn't have any trace of this genetic disease. I didn't say, "You, Hank, shall have an affliction that makes it hard to live." I was a mother; one who knew it wasn't a virus and was working on making him comfortable and healthy.

Any guilt I felt needed to go away – no one did this to him. It was the luck of genetics and, frankly, it doesn't matter how or why he has this disease. At the end of the day, he does have it.

Still, the guilt creeps in. It usually happens when Hank is having a flare; vomiting, refusing to eat, losing weight, acting out, crying in pain and feeling lethargic, and unable to sleep. Recognizing that the

RULE #2
lose the guilt

guilt has moved in allows me to act on it, and when this happens, I do the following:

1. First, I take myself out of the situation for a few moments. Even telling the children "Momma needs a time out" and then sitting alone and bringing myself back together, just for a few minutes, helps me regain my balance.

2. Next, I TALK. Talking to my husband and bouncing my thoughts off his often eradicates any fears or guilt I am feeling. It's an important lesson; you don't have to go through this alone.

There will always be times when you need to work on letting go of the guilt. It can and will eat you up if you don't. You need to be strong ... for yourself, and for your loved one. You have to be strong for the rest of the family too, who are dealing with their own often confusing and scary emotions.

Letting the guilt take you under is the surest way to surrender your strength.

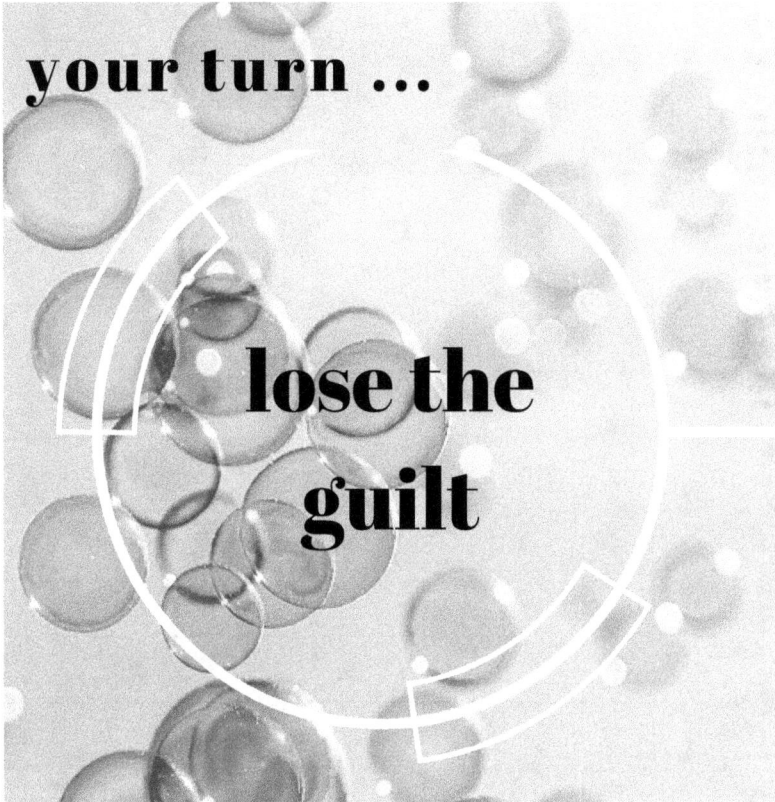

your turn ...

lose the guilt

THERE IS NO ROOM FOR GUILT, REMEMBER?

Yes, I just yelled at you; I am that serious about this. Yet I know as well as you do that it's hard to accept this and live this ... even when we know it's true. The key for me is recognizing when I start slipping into those guilt patterns. Recognizing it lets me act on it and pull myself out of the spiral. What triggers your feelings of guilt? How do you recognize it? And what can you do to pull yourself out of this unhelpful spiral? Write it all down on the next few pages, in all its gut-wrenching drama.

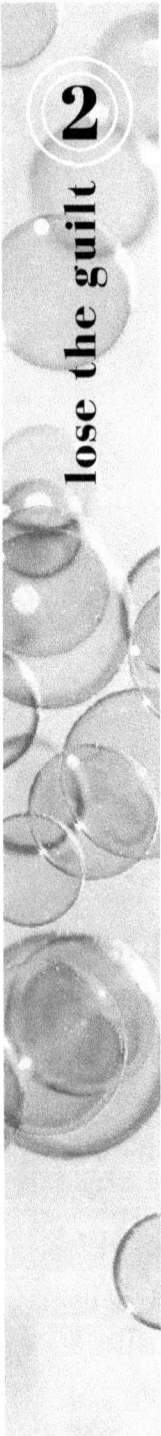

2

lose the guilt

date _____

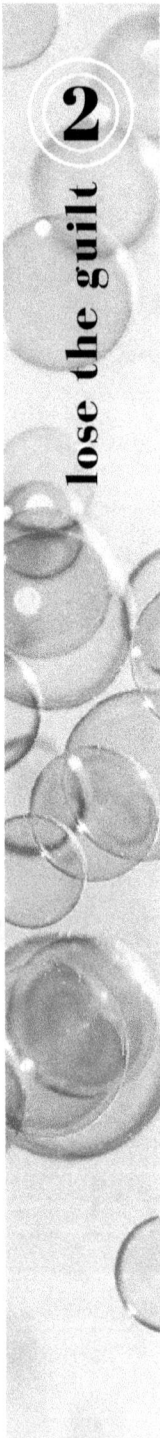

2

lose the guilt

date _____

date _____

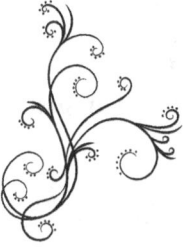

RULE #3
don't panic; get a plan

Still working full time and sending Hank to daycare while his brother started elementary school, I was living a massively hectic life. Scheduling doctor appointments, work schedules, elementary school homework and what was left of our family life had my husband and me not sleeping much and not thinking smart.

We took a critical look at my work life. I loved the work I did, but it was morphing into a stressful heap to try to manage it all. We decided it was time I resigned and stayed home. Our original plan was to maintain a daycare schedule but shorten the days. That worked for a while, until we found Hank's symptoms weren't clearing up and were in fact becoming worse; the allergen-free lunches I so carefully packed each day were not being served and, instead, Hank was being served... and eating ... the food he had already been reacting to!

His health was far more important than any educational or social benefits of hanging out with kids all day, so we removed him from the facility to stay at home with me. I began in earnest to learn how to cook for Hank, based on what we believed he could eat safely, with no reactions.

Being so sick so often from so many foods, he naturally developed a fear of eating. So, we catered to what he liked. We bought a deep fryer and I started making "Hank-Safe" chicken nuggets, and

31

RULE #3
don't panic; get a plan

continued to change the recipe when we found a new reaction. We learned, for instance, that tapioca flour makes an absolutely wonderful coating for the nuggets; it also caused Hank to want to scratch his skin off. It took another two years before we discovered it wasn't the tapioca causing the reaction, but the oil we used in the fryer. There were no more processed foods in Hank's diet, with the exception of the beloved Cheerios and one type of corn chip. Broccoli became a staple. Pulled pork was so successful with Hank that we bought our own smoker and regularly fill the neighborhood with smells so delicious we attract turkey vultures.

Even with all the uncertainty, we refused to panic. Because we didn't panic, we were able to think more clearly and get organized. We started planning menus around foods we could eat, finding ways to cook them so Hank would eat them. We had some failures, but with trial and error, and lots of deep breathing, we had several successes. Life became a little easier.

I learned the simple value of breathing deeply; taking myself out of the immediate situation helps center my thinking so I can focus on what needs to be done.

Talk to the people in your immediate circle of friends and family and share your fears and concerns. Then start making a plan together. How can you learn to work around the diagnosis? What changes can you make to help the situation? And how can the people around you help?

It may not be feasible to quit your job to take care of your loved one full time; every family's situation has its own set of challenges. Work with what you've got, and accept whatever help others are willing to

RULE #3
don't panic; get a plan

give. This can go a long way toward taking panic and turning it into a plan.

Think of these next few pages as the blueprint of your own situation and the beginnings of a plan for dealing with it. You may want to bring this blueprint to your doctor to walk through; this might help you both uncover even more options.

your turn ...

don't panic; get a plan

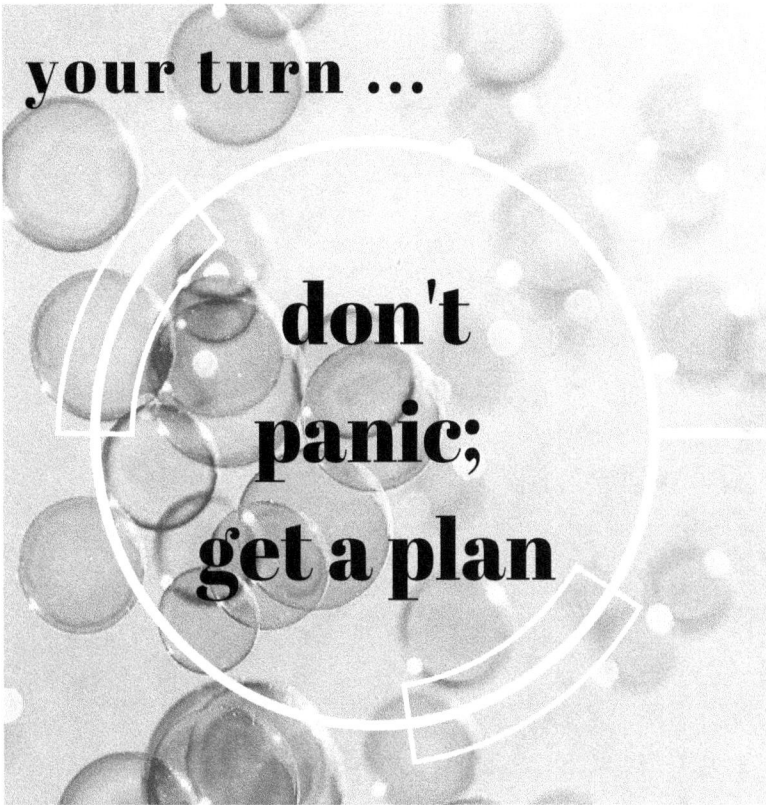

Start by writing down the situation as it is now. Include any day-to-day, week-to-week, month-to-month commitments and expectations. Then write down your ideas for moving ahead. Maybe you need to start planning menus, set up a med reminder system, or learn a new skill to help you through this path. (I learned oranges are a great way to practice using an EpiPen.) Finally, write down any tough issues and questions. Take your time with these pages, and jot down any possible solutions that spring to mind.

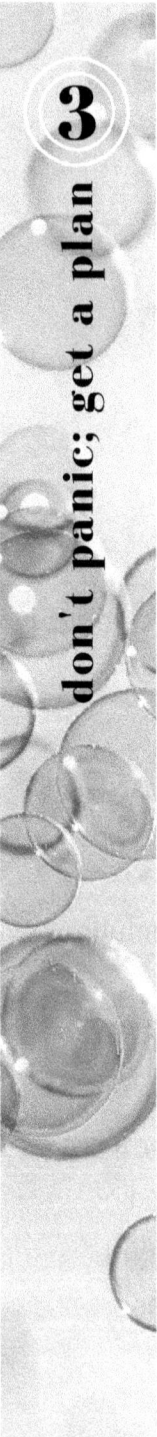

3

don't panic; get a plan

date _____

don't panic; get a plan

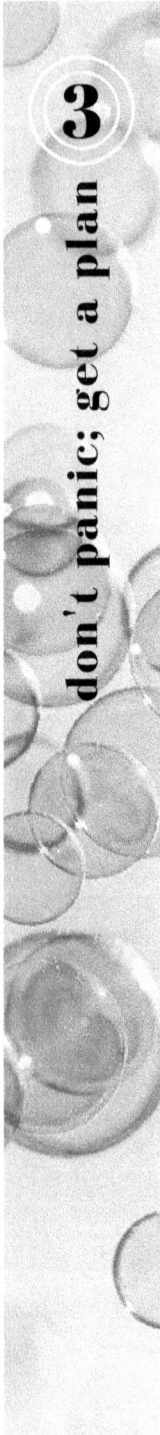

date _____

3

don't panic; get a plan

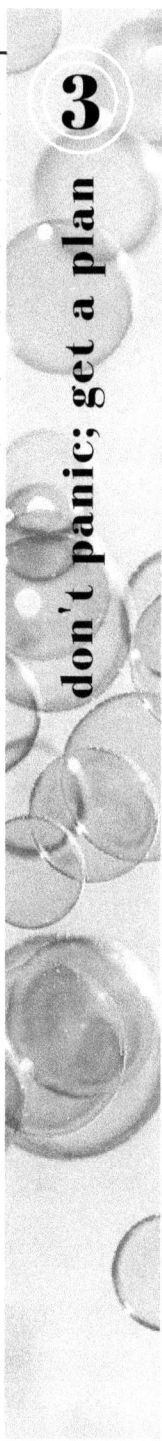

date _____

don't panic; get a plan

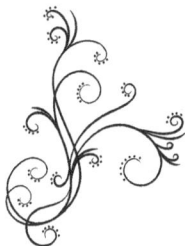

RULE #4
don't become a prisoner

There are days when I want to wallow … and I do. I keep Hank indoors all day and give in to his demands for juice and television. But I know in my heart that staying stagnant in the hope this will just go away isn't how life works.

For my son to be healthy, I need to concentrate on what we can do together and as a family to bring him to that state. But how do you teach a small child about life-threatening allergic reactions and how to avoid them, while leading some semblance of a "normal" life?

We talk. We talk a lot.

Just like we used flashcards to teach Hank his animals and numbers, we go over and over all the things he is allergic to. We don't want this to be a burden, but rather something so inherently a part of him, that it is, well, HIM — as much his as his blue eyes, left-handedness and Finnish stubbornness.

We went to our local library's story hour recently and one of his little friends was upset that I had not given Hank a snack to eat, but only a bottle of apple juice, so he offered Hank his own snack. I wasn't near them when this happened, but the other mothers sitting nearby told me that Hank stopped his friend and said, "No, I am allergic to that" and continued to happily drink his juice.

Just like that, Hank showed me this horrible disease wasn't

RULE #4
don't become a prisoner

going to hold him back. There was no drama, no angst, just matter of fact reality. It was then I realized that our diagnosis shouldn't hold us back.

Hank and I leave the house for museum field trips, zoo romps and story hours. I can't expect him to avoid normal interactions with the rest of the world because I'm afraid he will break. I need to look at what is best for this little boy and what is best for my sanity and not keep us pent up, prisoners in our home and our comfortably safe bubble. Obviously, do not discount what your doctor has said about the limitations of the condition you're dealing with. I'm careful not to over-run Hank when I know he hasn't taken in enough calories. Likewise, I don't let him sleep with the windows open at night when the hedges are in bloom. Still, we've found other ways of taking back our independence.

Finding a freedom of spirit can be as easy as painting Hank's toes before a scope, remembering our wacky sense of humor when we are talking to the nurses, or blowing bubbles outside in the middle of winter.

Living with a rare disease means you're forced to play by a lot of rules you didn't ask for; living well with a rare disease requires accepting those rules, then creating new rules that bring you joy, happiness, and a sense of freedom.

your turn ...

don't become a prisoner

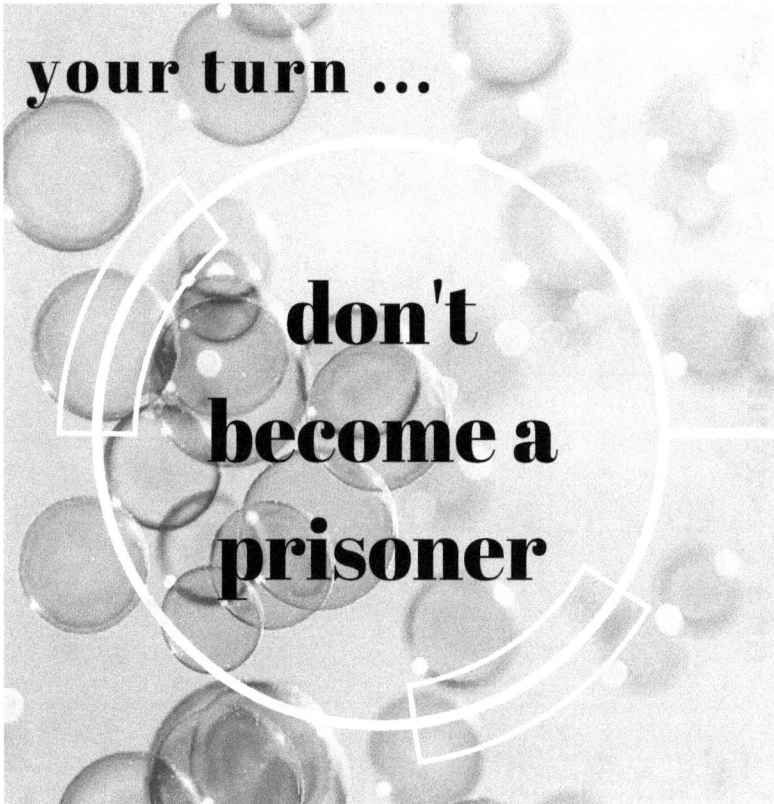

A rare diagnosis is not a lock on a jail cell. We've walked many a mile through a local museum, going weekly or sometimes more often. Sometimes we make a game of it, barricading the door to the living room and saying "we will not be shut in on the couch today!" What steps can you take to avoid becoming a prisoner to this disease? Use this space to find safe and simple ways you can regain a feeling of freedom.

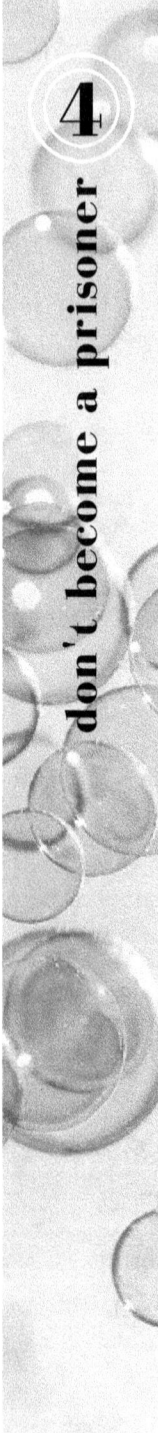

date _____

don't become a prisoner

date _____

don't become a prisoner

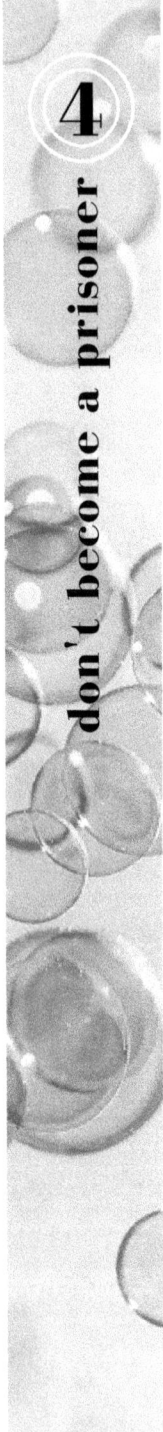

4

don't become a prisoner

date _____

don't become a prisoner

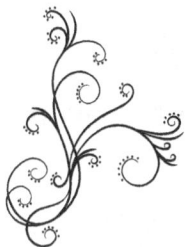

RULE #5
forward your thoughts

Even when I can keep the guilt away and stick to a plan, there are days when this is really tough. I am aware that my tough and someone else's tough can be on entirely different spectrums; still, I find that wading through it all is best done with a firm vision of the future, even if you can only look an hour, a day or a week ahead.

My looking forward might look something like this:

We're having a bad day.

Food isn't going in; reasoning with him isn't working ... so STOP.

He's likely in pain and isn't showing it.

If he spends today only drinking medical food or juice, TOMORROW he'll feel better, he'll be more comfortable, and he'll eat.

I had surgery myself last year. Sitting in the hospital bed post-op, I felt awful. I also had zero confidence I was going to feel better any time soon. But I stopped. I told myself yes, you feel awful now, but think about this time tomorrow. You will be feeling better, if only a bit. And this time the day after that, you will be feeling even better. I promise. And this time next week, you'll be walking and thinking how great you feel, and it just rolls on from there.

Looking forward helps us deal with the present because it gives

49

RULE #5
forward your thoughts

us a goal. It's not about ignoring the present; the first part of this process is to recognize the current pain, acknowledge it, even honor it, before looking ahead to improvements. Looking forward works because I am actively controlling myself and my feelings; I have told my brain to be prepared, promised it that things will be better soon. Maybe there is a heavy rain cloud on you today. It may be there tomorrow, or replaced by another one. But what about next week or the week after, what about this time next month or next year?

A pain-free life may not be in the forecast (is it in anyone's, really?) but can you at least picture yourself having a better handle on things, gaining a better understanding of the treatments, or maybe having a new coping strategy for the symptoms?

Consciously and actively envisioning goals for the future – even if that future is just an hour or two from now – will unconsciously push you into a better mental place as you plan for a better day.

your turn ...

forward your thoughts

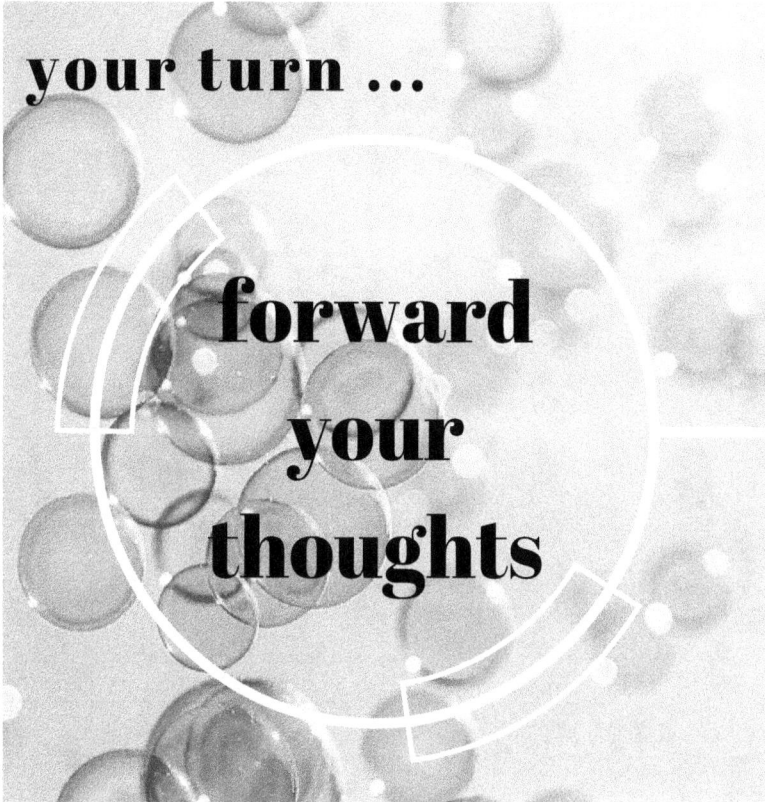

Start thinking about your personal goals. Maybe you have grand goals, like finally finding the right treatments to bring about a cure. Maybe your goal is as simple as making it through the next hour without shedding tears. In this section write down the goals you have today. Forward to tomorrow, next week, even next year. Make sure you date your entries; then you can return to this section later on and realize that today's hard situation is not tomorrow's.

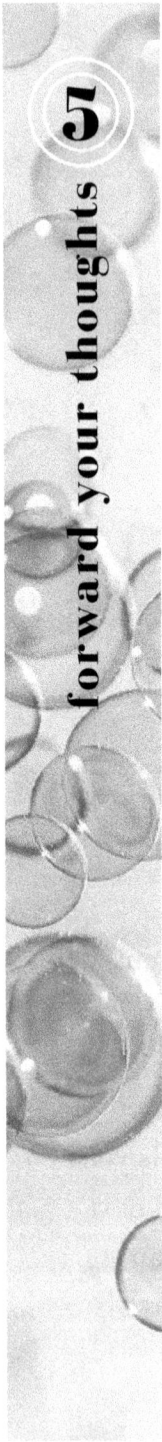

forward your thoughts

date _____

date _____

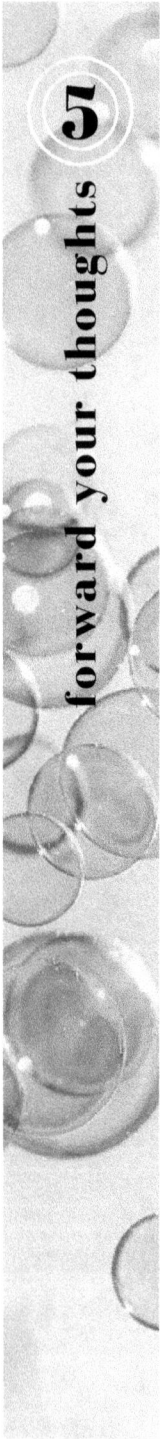

forward your thoughts

date _____

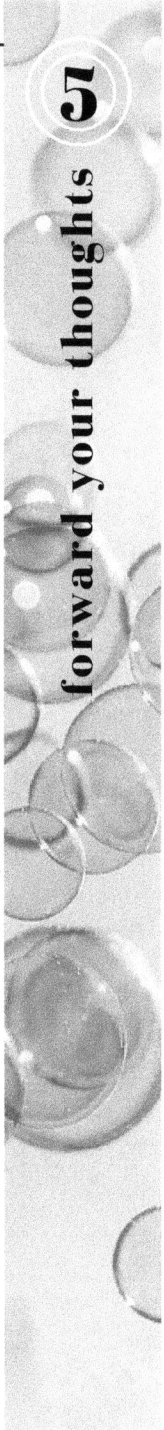

date _____

forward your thoughts

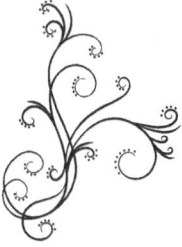

RULE #6
redefine normal

For families dealing with rare diseases, sometimes our normal isn't everyone's normal and that is OK. This is what I always tell my children about being different. If we were all the same, we would be boring and who wants to live in a boring world? I don't.

This life is our normal, and we've made it our own. We have pet names for his doctors (all of them have some sort of animal in their name). A trip to the emergency room after Daddy had a fall wasn't traumatic because we see the insides of hospitals regularly. Hank doesn't have a fear of needles, or doctors, or the strange sights and sounds there ... he's just afraid of food. Our normal means we paint Hank's toenails to entertain the nurses before each scope.

On the darker side of life, our normal also meant getting up multiple times a night for feedings through his seventh birthday. This IS our new normal.

Your normal may now be expensive medical food, sleepless nights and coffee rich mornings. Maybe it's endless loads of laundry, not being able to remember your last hair cut, or anything else that has begun to be a regular part of your life. You don't have to LIKE it, but the situation is your new normal.

Talk to your family and friends and explains to them how your

RULE #6
redefine normal

world is now different. This will help them understand what you're going through, and will help you better understand it too. Talking about it will make it real for everyone and, most importantly, you.

It's incredibly hard to move forward after a diagnosis stops you in your tracks. It's natural to resist the realities of the disease, and wish things were "back to normal." But ultimately that is a waste of time and energy. Instead, talk to your family and close friends about what's changed, and how your new normal impacts everything in your life. Once you understand the new normal caused by the diagnosis, you can begin to make the changes that will reinvent normal once again in ways you can control. Redefining normal is not easy, but it's been one of the most effective things I've done for our family.

Our lives are different with the reality of dealing with this disease, but we accept and embrace that it is our life. For Hank, it is the only normal he knows. For the rest of us in our little family, we remind ourselves that eating out, traveling and even our kitchen now has a different look — and it is perfectly okay. It is our new normal.

your turn ...

redefine normal

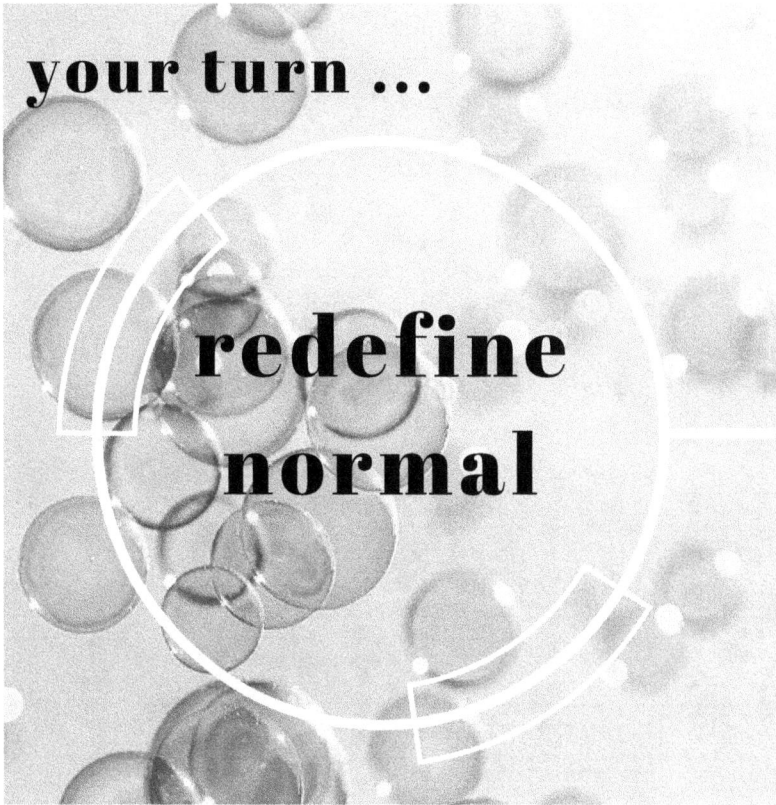

What's changing in your life due to this disease? What will be "normal" for you now? Write down the new realities and embrace them; this is your life. This is your new normal.

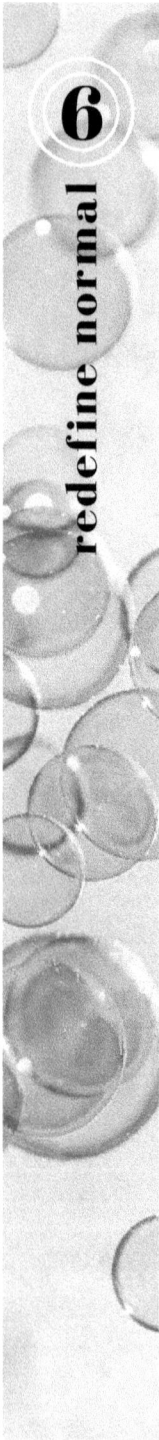

redefine normal

date _____

date _____

redefine normal

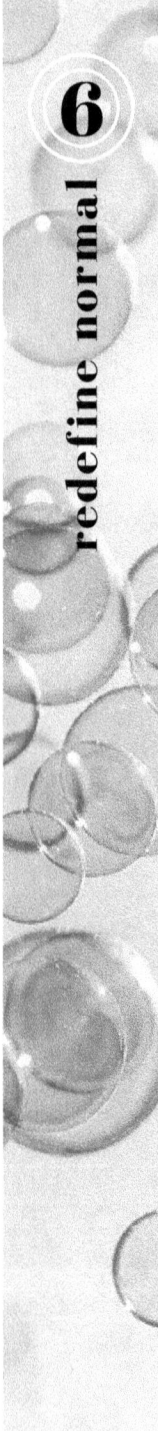

6

redefine normal

date _____

redefine normal

Wendy Price

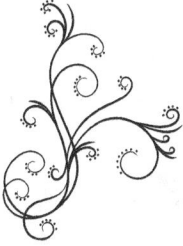

RULE #7
seek out others

When we received Hank's mind-numbing diagnosis, I heard the word "RARE." I focused on that, assuming we were the only family in our town, our state, our universe dealing with this thing called EoE. I felt incredibly alone.

So I reached out to the internet and whoa! I found social media groups FULL of parents who have children, some even multiple children, with EoE. I found moms and dads sharing stories about keeping up with formula, meals, trading recipes, sharing strategies for dealing with school, work, family life …

Suddenly, we were no longer alone. Not even close. Less than five miles from our home, we learned of a high school senior with EoE; his mom had been diligently documenting his struggles with their local high school. As a community, we all celebrated when he graduated on time and with honors, even though he had missed a ton of school due to flare-ups.

When we enrolled Hank into kindergarten, he was one of three kids with EoE at his school! He was definitely not alone.

I've been in the black void, where you feel no one can possibly get what you're going through. Yet please remember this: No matter how alone you feel, you are not alone in this experience. As devastating as this blow can be to our hearts, emotions and souls, there is almost

65

RULE #7
seek out others

always someone feeling the exact same thing that you are. Seek them out through hospital support groups, social workers or Facebook Groups.

As a habit, I don't share too much publicly on the Facebook boards, but I read what others write and I respond to them, reaching out to them with gratitude and compassion. Doing so has put this diagnosis into clear perspective. I have come to realize there are others with this disease who have it worse than Hank. I take in their stories and their suggestions, and offer my own thoughts when I see a topic that we've gone through in our family.

Hank, being seven now, doesn't have a cell phone or his own computer; he doesn't really have a grasp on what social media is all about. Still, I will often show him pictures from the people I've connected with, showing children getting ready for scopes, celebrating when they pass a new food, offering support when they've failed a food, sharing their anxiety when their child gets a feeding tube.

This is our community of warriors; we are all fighting the same battles. We need a tribe on our side, a group of people who understand the stakes of this battle. When Hank was first diagnosed with EoE, his allergist suggested a few websites and social media groups for me to check out. He wanted me to learn more about this disease, but he also knew how important it would be for me and our family to connect with others who are living with EoE.

As new allergies, poor growth, and weird flares have popped up (which they seemed to do with alarming frequency), these online social groups have truly been a lifesaver. Suggestions and conversations on what has worked for others have given us new ways of

RULE #7
seek out others

thinking forward, and confirmed that we do not have to face this alone.

Seek out your tribe. Friends are important, but you need to connect with others who truly understand what you are dealing with. Ask for recommendations from your doctor, and actively seek out those who will understand and ultimately give you an additional sounding board. As you seek this out, figure out how your other interests can help you relate to your new normal.

For example, I always loved to bake and cook before we had food restrictions in our kitchen. Thanks to these groups, I have found boards that cater to baking and cooking with EoE, so I can still enjoy something that brings me joy, while keeping everything Hank-safe. There's a real bonus to this; what I've learned on one board carries over to another, so I can contribute my own ideas on safe recipes and creative adaptations. My new normal may be different, certainly, but it still tastes sweet. I couldn't have gotten to this point without the compassionate help of so many others going through similar challenges.

your turn ...

seek out others

Where can you find others going through a similar experience? Take some time now and research some groups, then connect on social media and use the following pages to note the groups you've joined. Keep adding to the list as you join more. (And make sure to connect with @10 Little Rules on Facebook and Twitter, and @10 Little Rules of Hank on Facebook and Instagram. You're always welcome there, and I can supply more information on safe places to connect with other EOE families.)

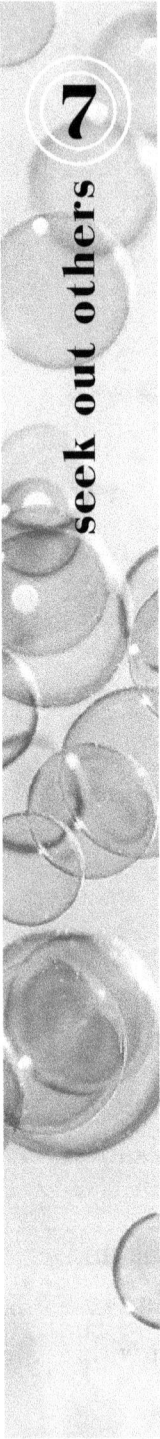

7

seek out others

date _____

seek out others

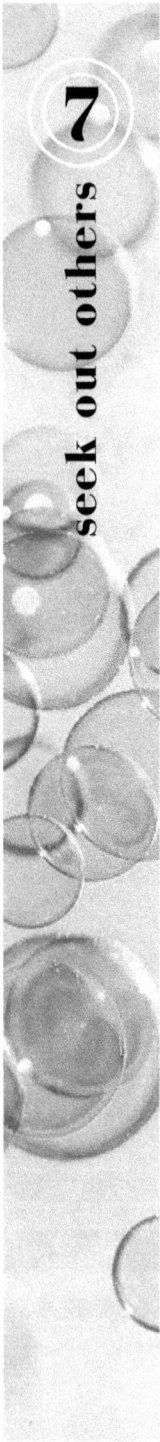

seek out others

date _____

date _____

seek out others

7

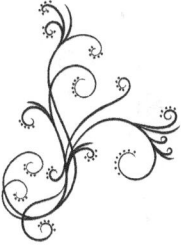

RULE #8
embrace the humor

Life with a rare disease is tense; it is serious. When you are dealing with a rare disease, spraying down your oldest child with shaving cream is sometimes a necessity. Sending crazy selfies of yourself to your working spouse can be a highlight of your day.

What is it about being funny that takes the weight off our shoulders? Laughing is as therapeutic as crying, maybe even more so. I know from experience that my head aches after a fit of crying. But my soul is brighter after just a few moments of laughing. I know which I would rather do to release the stress.

There is a vision I have in my brain on reserve. When things seem really dark, I think of this summertime memory. The four of us filled large balloons with water and took them into the front yard. The water fight got intense, pretty quickly. Once my husband was thoroughly drenched, he picked up an enormous balloon and aimed it at Dave. He got him square in the back … it LAUNCHED him three feet, right into the flower bed. He was shocked, but safe and unhurt. And I couldn't stop laughing. Dave's revenge on his father led to more splashes, laughter and joy. That was a lovely day.

Serious illness or not, my kids are kids and they behave accordingly. There are times when their bickering and fighting have me at my wits' end. There are times when Hank picks on his big

RULE #8
embrace the humor

brother Dave; my older son can't really defend himself, seeing how tiny his brother is.

At times like this I tell them: "Stop fighting / bickering / nagging / talking or I will trade you for goats." Invariably, this leads to a hilarious discussion of how big the goats would have to be for a fair trade. Or silly chatter about what I would have the goats do. That one's easy, I tell them. They would eat my lawn so I don't have to mow. But what will I do if I get tired of the goats? Ask them that question and both boys will tell you, "She's going to eat them!"

Redirecting a tense situation or a bad day with humor is such a wonderful way to get through life, no matter what you are facing. A word of caution, however: I have found it's quite rare to find an anesthesiologist who thinks you are as funny as you believe you are. No humor there, I'll tell you. I keep trying.

Humor has an incredible power to take the edge off a tense situation, and let our minds relax for a bit. It lifts our hearts, and shows us that our new normal can be satisfying and indeed joyful.

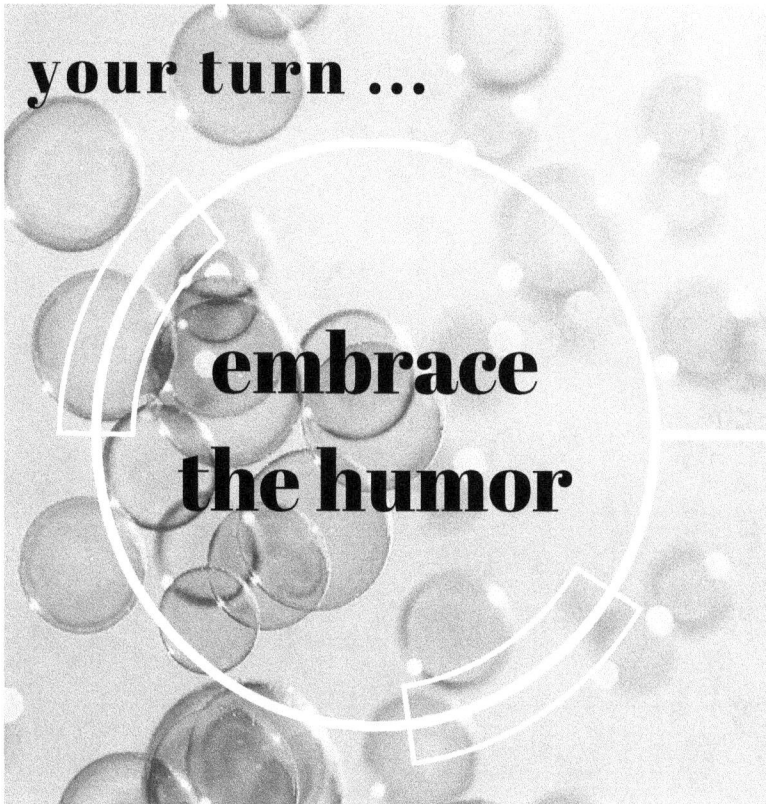

your turn ...

embrace the humor

What makes you laugh? Silly cat videos? Fart humor? (I have two boys; I hear a lot of fart talk.) The goat farm? Think of a few things recently that made you laugh, smile or simply feel good. Write them down on the following pages. Come back to these pages often and add to the list. The more you write down, the more you'll start seeing the humor all around us.

date _____

embrace the humor

date _____

enbrace the humor

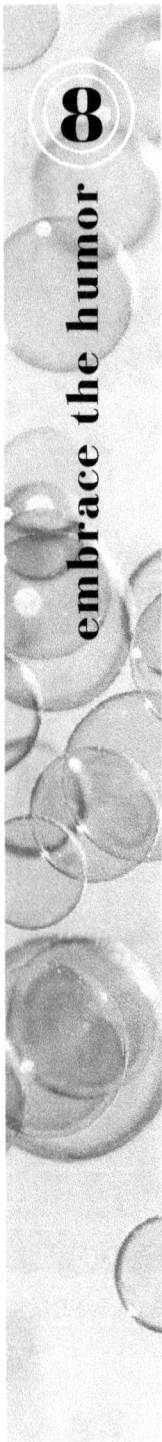

8

embrace the humor

date _____

embrace the humor

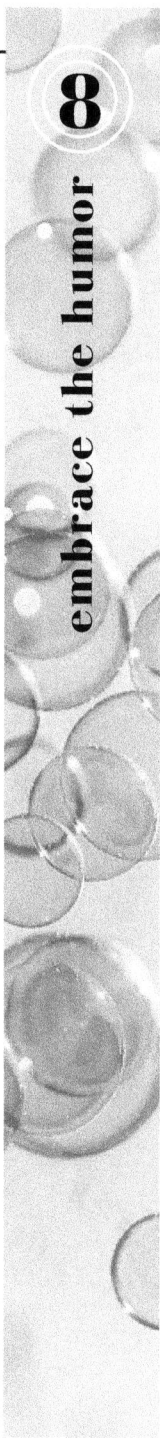

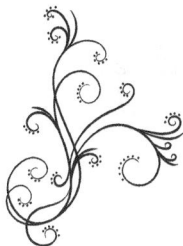

RULE #9
make it better

In Rule 10, I am going to tell you to give thanks. Yet, I can already hear you asking:

"Thanks? For what? Why? Everything that could be wrong is wrong and nothing is going to make it better!"

I hear you, I really do. But remember Rule 5? Think Forward. Will tomorrow be better? Yes, because you can make it better. And Rule 6, Redefine Normal. I know this can be a tough one; redefining our normal forces us to accept that life with this disease is a permanent thing. Yet, once you begin to lean into those two rules you will be well on your way to making the situation better. Look for the silver lining in your day – it's there, even if it's just a tiny glint at first.

The disease may be outside your control, but your life is still your own. You can let yourself fall into a pit of despair, or you can work on living life happily. For me, I try to compliment at least one person a day – their shoes, clothing, their children's manners may catch my eye and I don't hesitate to comment on it. It's so important to know that everything in this world can start with you and your view of it. This simple act can change someone else's day for the better, and that in turn can make you happier. It's really that simple.

If, at the end of the day, I still haven't passed out a compliment – guess who gets it? I do!

RULE #9
make it better

I made it through the day without having a tantrum!

I made dinner for the family and some percentage of the folks around the table decided it was edible enough to eat without dying!

I finally called the air conditioner folks to schedule that checkup! GOOD FOR ME!! I've done a good job.

Another ritual I have is to name a "person of the day." This one can get a little strange, and really fun. Maybe I see something amazing on Instagram and that person has blown my mind and is now my person of the day. That person might not know me, may never know me, but their action shone a light into my day.

A dear friend of mine mentioned how far she lived from work; construction was making it harder and her commute was well over an hour. I didn't really think too much about it, as we all have to drive to work, but I had to run her route one day in rush hour and I realized just how much further she had to drive than probably anyone else in the office. I sent her a message when I got home and told her that I understood how far she had to drive every day just so I could see her face at work and therefore, she was my person of the day because I appreciated her.

By deciding for yourself each day what's great, even awesome, you take back some control in a very positive way. You get to decide what's good in your day, and focus on that. It's a really powerful way to change your day for the better.

When you find those silver linings, write them down. Consider keeping a separate journal where you can jot your notes. This is one entry from mine:

RULE #9
make it better

Hank has not eaten at all this week.

He has only nibbled through meals, hidden his snacks AND threw away his lunch at school.

But ...

Hank communicated to me that he wasn't feeling well.

Hank wanted to help make dinner.

Hank says that he loves me.

This isn't about measuring and recording leaps and bounds; it is simply looking at the bad and countering them with the good. This helps you move on further in understanding and acceptance.

Some days I do have to force myself to look for the silver lining and the good in life. Other days it comes easy. Every day, it is there; it's up to you to find it and take it.

your turn ...

make it better

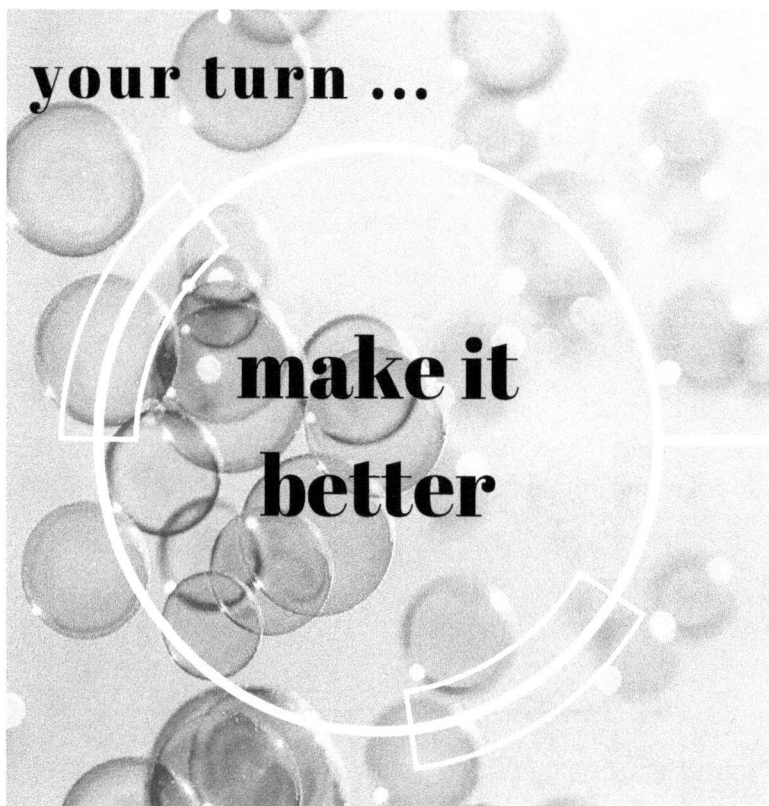

What is the absolute worst thing about your new normal? Write it down on the following pages. Then take a critical look. Is it permanent? It could be, or maybe the silver lining is that it's better today than it was yesterday. Take a closer look at your new normal. What's the best part of it? Have you connected with others, or found support in an unlikely place? Have you discovered strengths or talents you didn't know you had? Make note of all the silver linings peeking out from behind those clouds.

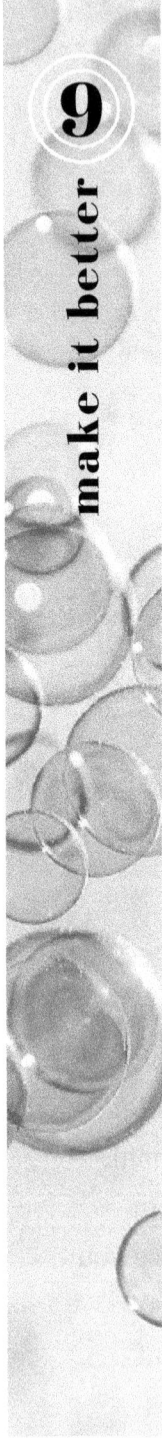

9

make it better

date _____

make it better

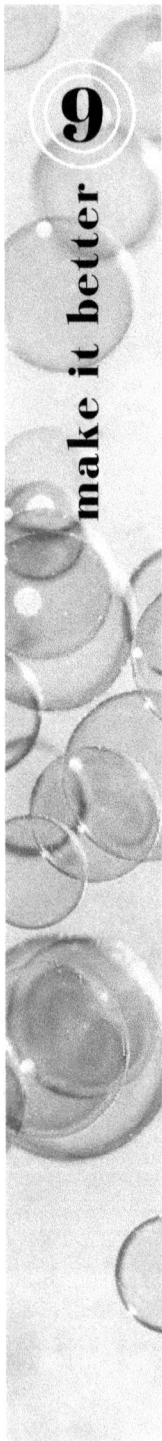

9

make it better

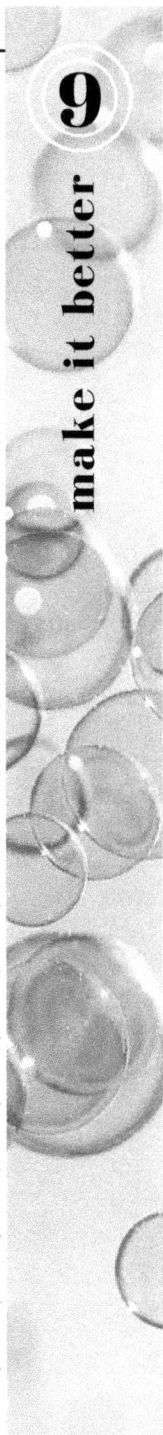

date _____

make it better

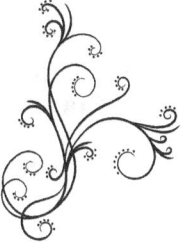

RULE #10
every day, give thanks

Take some time for yourself every day. Mine is usually right as my husband is putting the kids to bed. Those glorious 15 minutes, when Dave is reading to himself and Hank is drinking his final cup of medical food, is my time to reflect on the day. I weed through the actions of each child and think about what is growing, maturing or just normal kid behavior. Then I mentally begin to reset my mind from the day to the evening and in turn for the day ahead.

I think about the good things that happened that day, the bad things, and what could have been worse. I take this time to affirm that the next day is new and everything will reset overnight and we'll start anew in the early hours of the next morning. And I am thankful for that.

I am thankful for my children; their love, their differences, how alike they are and how happy (and sometimes frustrated) they make me.

Was your day especially hairy? What was your silver lining? Nothing? I've had my share of days where I believed that to be true.

On those days, I simply thank myself for making it through the day in one piece. Be thankful that the sun came out and you saw it – or be thankful that it came out and you stood in it and blocked that energy from touching the earth. You controlled the sun and it had

RULE #10
every day, give thanks

to shine on you instead.

You are fierce and powerful, and you've got this.

You've written down some hard stuff so far; diving into this is not easy work. You've had to come to grips with your new normal, let go of any guilt you've been harboring and start asking others for help. THIS rule is simple, though. Just give thanks. You are here, you have opened your mind to a new way of getting through this, and you have a plan of action to help you move forward on your journey.

The simple act of gratitude, finding things each day for which we are truly grateful, is the secret to finding new strength and new courage to face your new normal. It is the secret to staying positive in the midst of so much you cannot control. And while this rule might sound simple, I know it may not be easy. So I'll help you out by starting with this:

Thank you, YOU.

YOU are the person of the day.

You read my silly little book, you learned a bit about me and I know you'll find some way to let my thoughts help ease your situation.

Keep being awesome!

your turn ...

every day, give thanks

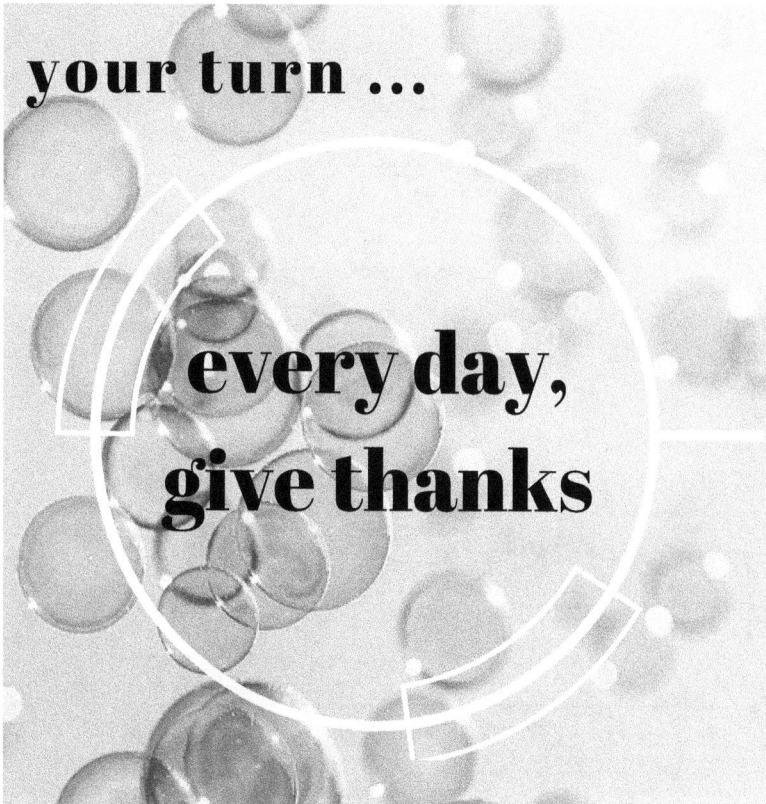

What are you thankful for, right now? Be serious, be silly, be profound or be goofy, but be authentic. What are you grateful for, right now? Write down anything that crosses your mind. Come back to these pages often to add to the list. As you make gratitude a habit, this rule becomes the ground on which you'll stand.

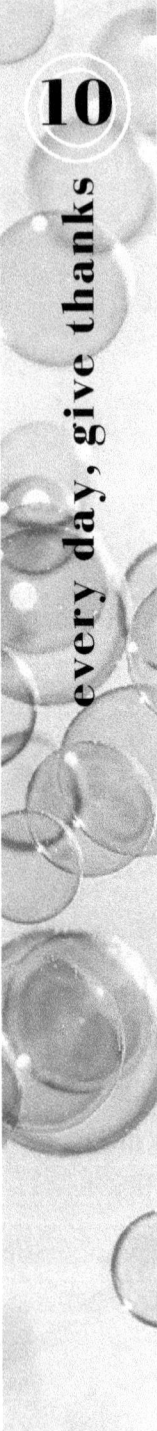

every day, give thanks

date _____

date _____

every day, give thanks

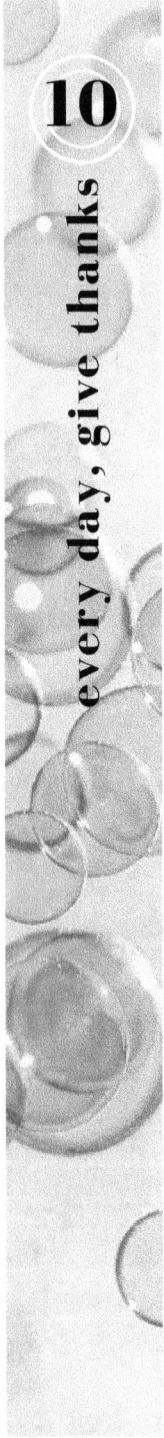

10

every day, give thanks

date _____

date _____

every day, give thanks

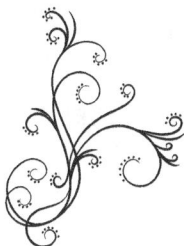

RULE #11?
carry on...

So, um, 10 Little Rules and here I am, throwing in one more?! Do I really have more to say or am I getting paid by the word? Or am I just an over-achiever?

This is the fun part: There is no end. None. Just when you think you have the situation under control, life throws something else at you. How do you handle it? How do you read through all these rules and do the work and think you're getting things sorted out and now it is all upside down? What then?

The truth is you will never have life all figured out. If we did, it would be so boring. Sure, relapses, big medical procedures and even bigger medical bills aren't exciting, at least in the fun way – but they're certainly not boring!

Some of these wrenches in life are easy to see coming, sometimes they are not. We have a BIG one coming up. As much of this book was being written, it was summer vacation for my older child; he went into 4th grade and Hank was about to start all-day kindergarten; with other kids, foods, hands that may not have been fully washed and situations that he has just never been in. My carefully controlled normal was about to get a dose of real-world reality. These germs gave me a new reason to lose sleep at night.

When life comes knocking, I've found making plans is the best

RULE #11

carry on

way to start. You know you have a situation where you may need to explain your reality to others. Making sure that you have a plan makes a world of difference.

I knew that we were about to try public school, so I put together a plan. We met with the principal of Hank's soon-to-be-elementary school and the district's nurse. I had already scoured my Facebook groups for the information I was going to need, and was given an incredibly helpful document from another mother that she had put together for her child. I followed her format, changed it to reflect Hank's situation and even remembered to change out the "she's" to "he's." I had it all ready for his first day, to help the team at school understand Hank and his needs.

Something as simple as a card in your wallet with some important information can help you feel more in control: an explanation of the diagnosis, the location of any emergency medications, and contact info of a trusted friend, all these things will help when you find yourself in a panicky situation. Does your child have a long list of medications? Print or write them out on one side of a card, with your doctors' names, specialties and numbers on the other. Update this card as needed, and keep it with you. Make a copy and keep it on the fridge or post it somewhere that family can access it if you're not home.

I also recommend sitting down with your trusted circle of family and friends to discuss various emergency possibilities and how you would like them handled. Make sure your doctor understands these needs and your wishes as well.

We can't be prepared for everything. There is just no way to know what will happen next. But we can be prepared with the information we'll need; this could definitely help diffuse some of the panic from a

RULE #11
carry on

situation that is likely already frantic.

As I write this, we're now roughly halfway through Hank's second year in school. I cannot plan for all the illnesses that come with mixing so many kids together, but I now have a better idea of what we are facing this year. I know that careful planning, and focusing on our new normal, is how we'll get through.

Carrying on means more than simply getting through the next obstacle or emergency. It means reevaluating everything, trying new avenues of treatment. It means finding new ways of living and new ways of thinking.

For Hank and our family, we continue to think forward. We have recently changed healthcare providers, and Hank has undergone another endoscopy.

Our new normal? We are now in REMISSION. *Cue the confetti and balloons falling from the ceiling while a big band plays Hank's favorite Twisted Sister song, as we dance with champagne glasses filled with mango juice!*

Remission, in Hank's case, means the biopsy of his esophagus came back with no significant traces of eosinophils. He still has this disease; these results simply mean it's not active at the moment. His weight still hovers around the 3rd percentile, so something has to change – we've gone back onto medical foods, and trying some new foods. With a clear scope and little weight gain, we have decided to go back and reevaluate his allergens. Initially we had removed so many foods, based on testing that is ultimately non-conclusive, that there may have been foods that were caught in the cross fire but aren't true allergens for Hank.

With a watchful eye for vomiting and other symptoms, we're

RULE #11
carry on

starting an eight-week challenge of adding soy and egg into our diets. If Hank passes this, wonderful. If not, then we remove those foods again and continue on to tackle the next allergen in question.

Wish us luck; we may have nights of flares and vomits in our near future. Yet every "yes" food is one more silver lining in our new normal. So we carry on.

As for you, know that our family wishes you luck too as you navigate your way through a rare disease. We wish you strength and peace, humor and giggles, and so much support as you carry on.

We are all in this together.

your turn ...

carry on

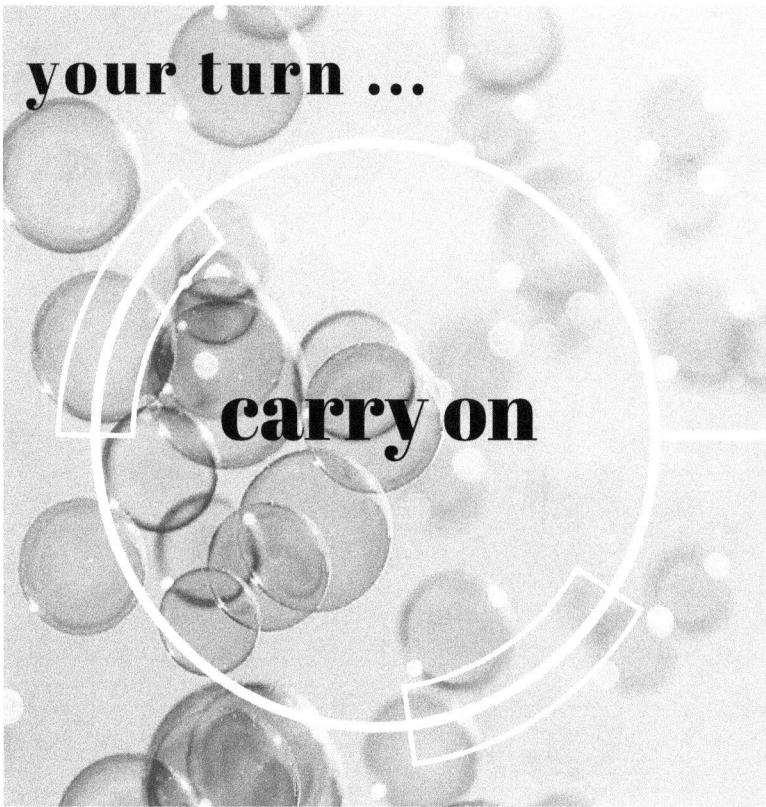

Is there an ugly fear lurking just on the edge of your mind? Is there any confusion about this illness or your new normal? Take a moment to confront the fear, face the confusion, and embrace the mystery of your new life. You can't move forward without being able to fully accept your situation. Use these next pages to get it all out.

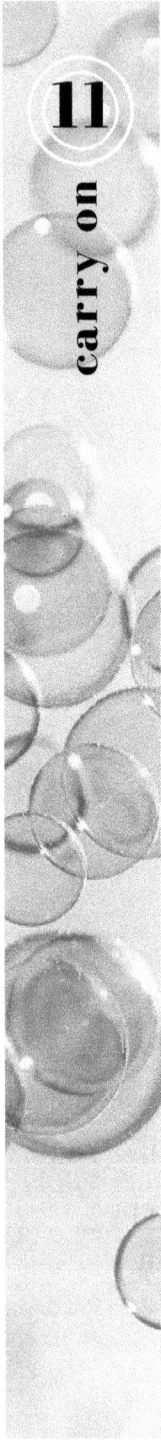

11

carry on

date _____

carry on

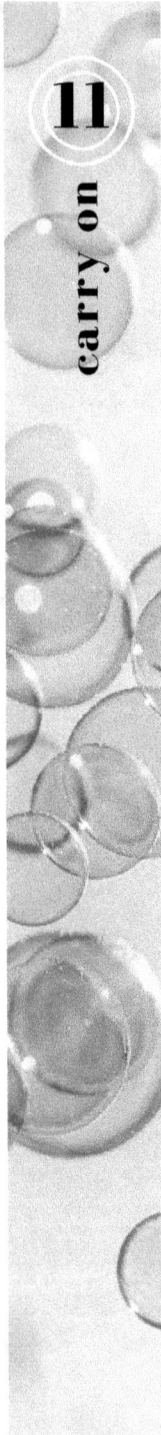

carry on

date _____

date _____

carry on

10 LITTLE RULES
connect with our community

Stay connected to
the 10 Little Rules Community

Like and Follow our Facebook
page at facebook.com/10LittleRules
for ongoing support and discussion on
how to apply these books to living your best life.

For updates on Hank and support for the journey through a
rare disease, follow his Instagram
@10_little_rules_of_hank

Visit our website for updates at www.10littlerules.com

Books in the 10 Little Rules series:
10 Little Rules for a Blissy Life by Carol Pearson
10 Little Rules for Your Creative Soul by Rita Long
10 Little Rules of Hank by Wendy Price

Watch for more 10 Little Rules books launching soon!

www.ingramcontent.com/pod-product-compliance
Lightning Source LLC
Chambersburg PA
CBHW062103270326
41931CB00013B/3190